Preface

The Infant Feeding Survey has been conducted every five years since 1975 and captures a wealth of information about infant feeding practices in the United Kingdom. It helps to describe historical trends in infant feeding practice and identify opportunities for improved implementation of national policy. The Scientific Advisory Committee on Nutrition (SACN) Subgroup on Maternal and Child Nutrition (SMCN) has reviewed the findings of the 2005 Infant Feeding Survey. It particularly welcomes the significant increases observed in breastfeeding initiation across the UK and a marked reduction in the proportion of infants given solid foods at an inappropriately young age.

This review recommends options to improve infant feeding practice and informs infant feeding policy. It also suggests areas for deeper exploration in future quinquennial surveys, particularly to take account of the national implementation of "Healthy Start" in 2006 and to define its effects on practice.

SACN wishes to draw attention to the fundamental importance of this area of public health nutrition. I welcome this report and thank all members of the Subgroup for their time and valued contribution.

Professor Alan Jackson
Chair of the Scientific Advisory Committee on Nutrition
January 2008

Contents

Membership of Scientific Advisory Committee on Nutrition: Subgroup on Maternal and Child Nutrition (SMCN):

Chairman:

Dr Anthony F Williams — Reader in Child Nutrition & Consultant in Neonatal Paediatrics, St George's University of London

Members:

Professor Peter Aggett — Head of School, Lancashire School of Health and Medicine, Professor of Child Health and Nutrition, University of Central Lancashire

Professor Annie S Anderson — Professor of Food Choice, Centre for Public Health Nutrition Research, University of Dundee

Dr Robert Fraser — Reader, Reproductive and Developmental Medicine, University of Sheffield

Professor Alan A Jackson — Professor of Human Nutrition, Southampton General Hospital

Professor Timothy Key — Professor in Epidemiology, University of Oxford Cancer Research UK Epidemiology Unit, Radcliffe Infirmary, Oxford

Dr Ann Prentice — Director, Medical Research Council Human Nutrition Research, Cambridge

Mrs Stella M Walsh — Senior Lecturer, Leeds Metropolitan University

Observers:

Rosemary Hignett	Food Standards Agency
Fiona Bisset	Scottish Government, Health Department
Maureen Howell	The Welsh Assembly, Health Promotion Division
Naresh Chada	Department of Health, Social Services and Public Safety, Northern Ireland
Rachel Atkinson	Department of Health

Secretariat:

Dr Sheela Reddy (Scientific)

Rachel Coomber (Scientific)

Membership of Scientific Advisory Committee on Nutrition (SACN):

Chairman:

Professor Alan A Jackson

Professor of Human Nutrition, Southampton General Hospital

Members:

Professor Peter Aggett

Head of School, Lancashire School of Health and Medicine, Professor of Child Health and Nutrition, University of Central Lancashire

Professor Annie S Anderson

Professor of Food Choice, Centre for Public Health Nutrition Research, University of Dundee

Professor Sheila Bingham

Director, Medical Research Council Centre for Nutrition and Cancer Prevention and Survival. Group Leader, Medical Research Council's Dunn Human Nutrition Unit, Cambridge

Mrs Christine Gratus

Retired Director and International Vice-President of J Walter Thompson Advertising Agency (lay member)

Dr Paul Haggarty

Senior Research Scientist at Rowett Research Institute.

Honorary clinical scientist NHS Trust

Professor Timothy Key

Professor in Epidemiology, University of Oxford

Cancer Research UK Epidemiology Unit, Radcliffe Infirmary, Oxford

Professor Peter Kopelman

Professor of Clinical Medicine, Vice-Principal/Deputy Warden (Education). Barts and The London, Queen Mary's School of Medicine and Dentistry, University of London

Professor Ian Macdonald

Professor of Metabolic Physiology, University of Nottingham. Director of Research at the Faculty of Medicine and Health Sciences

Dr David Mela	Senior Scientist and Expertise Group Leader, Unilever Food and Health Research Institute (Industry member)
Dr Ann Prentice	Director, Medical Research Council Human Nutrition Research, Cambridge
Dr Anita Thomas	Associate Medical Director / Consultant Physician in General (Internal) and Geriatric Medicine, Derriford Hospital, Plymouth Hospitals NHS Trust Clinical Sub Dean, Peninsula Medical School, Universities of Exeter and Plymouth
Mrs Stella M Walsh	Senior Lecturer, Leeds Metropolitan University
Dr Anthony F Williams	Reader in Child Nutrition & Consultant in Neonatal Paediatrics, St George's University of London

Observers:

Rosemary Hignett	Food Standards Agency
Fiona Bisset	Scottish Government, Health Department
Maureen Howell	The Welsh Assembly, Health Promotion Division
Naresh Chada	Department of Health, Social Services and Public Safety, Northern Ireland
Rachel Atkinson	Department of Health

Secretariat:

Dr Sheela Reddy (Scientific)

Rachel Coomber (Scientific)

Dr Elaine Stone (Scientific)

Executive Summary

1. Promoting and supporting optimal maternal and infant nutrition is important, particularly among population groups where breastfeeding rates are low. Breastmilk is the optimal diet for infants, and research continues to strengthen this position, notably in relation to the health risks attributable to not breastfeeding.

2. The latest Infant Feeding Survey was conducted in 2005 and is the seventh survey of its type. It provides national estimates of breastfeeding incidence and prevalence as well as capturing data on other aspects of infant feeding, such as the use of breastmilk substitutes and information about weaning practices. In addition, the survey collects information about the type and quality of antenatal and postnatal support available for pregnant and breastfeeding mothers. The survey thus identifies potential strengths and weaknesses that exist in the implementation of current infant feeding policy, uncovering for attention those areas in which mothers lack support.

3. Government policy in the United Kingdom has consistently promoted breastfeeding as a desirable population norm and in addition to UK wide strategies, specific approaches have been developed in England, Scotland, Wales and Northern Ireland to support breastfeeding and encourage good infant feeding practices.

4. The survey showed that breastfeeding rates have increased since the 2000 survey. It was also the first to identify the proportion of mothers exclusively breastfeeding. Breastfeeding rates were affected by the mothers' awareness of the health benefits of breastfeeding, antenatal care and postnatal support received, problems experienced with breastfeeding, peer influences and also when the mother returned to work.

5. Key findings from the survey highlight the inequalities in infant feeding that still exist and there is a consistent pattern of practices associated with socio-demographic characteristics of the mother. Young mothers and mothers from lower socio-economic groups appear to be the least likely to adopt infant feeding practices recommended by Health Departments.

6. A significant increase in the proportion of mothers appropriately delaying the introduction of solids was observed in the 2005 survey. This is an encouraging

move forward, which indicates that advice is successfully reaching mothers. Few mothers actually delayed introduction of solids until the recommended time of six months, suggesting a need to promote this message more widely. The time at which mothers introduced solids appeared largely to be affected by professional support and guidance received.

7. The proportion of mothers using infant formula as the sole source of nutrition for their baby from birth, was lower than in 2000. The survey also showed a high proportion of mothers using follow-on formula and giving additional drinks such as juice and water at an early age, despite advice that there is no nutritional justification for this. It appears mothers are not consistently aware of advice that breastmilk is the only food and drink an infant needs until the age of six months. The survey also raised concern about the preparation of formula; a large proportion of mothers were not following national guidance for safe preparation and storage of infant formula.

8. Despite recommendations from UK Health Departments regarding the use of vitamin supplements by pregnant or breastfeeding women and their infants, a large proportion of women were not taking supplements during pregnancy and lactation. An even larger proportion of mothers were not giving their babies vitamin supplements as recommended.

9. Actions required to improve policy implementation include:

- Raising awareness of the health risks associated with not breastfeeding and encouraging discussion of infant feeding during pregnancy, tailoring advice to social circumstances.

- Encouraging further delay in the introduction of solids to around six months of age. There is a need to alter the labelling of commercial weaning foods to reflect this advice.

- Making antenatal and postnatal services more accessible for hard-to-reach groups and encouraging them to use these services more frequently.

- Facilitating both hospital and community environments so that they are conducive to breastfeeding and ensuring that infant feeding advice and support are widely available and accessible to those who require it.

- Encouraging all health care providers to adopt the principles of UNICEF's Baby Friendly Initiative to actively encourage breastfeeding, with the aim of increasing both initiation and continuation rates.

- Ensuring that all health professionals receive adequate training in the practical management of breastfeeding support and that this is maintained. In addition, ensuring there are sufficient numbers of trained individuals to provide practical breastfeeding support.

- Encouraging provision of adequate infant feeding facilities in both the work place and in public places, to ensure these are available for those who require them.

- Clarifying and emphasising professional advice on the use of infant formula and follow-on formula, and encouraging the restriction of all forms of marketing communication.

- Ensuring that appropriate independent professional advice is provided to parents who choose to formula feed, to ensure that it is undertaken as safely as possible.

- Encouraging uptake of vitamins by both pregnant and breastfeeding women, and their infants, raising the importance of vitamin supplementation for these women and children, and particularly encouraging the uptake of Healthy Start vitamins.

- Raising the profile of Healthy Start, and offering practical support and advice to those eligible for the scheme.

- Implementing forthcoming NICE guidance for primary care on Maternal and Child Nutrition in low-income families.

10.   In addition, it is recommended that future surveys collect information on:

- Help and advice available to mothers throughout antenatal and postnatal care: and the forms of advice mothers find most useful and effective.

- The numbers of babies born in Baby Friendly hospitals, the stage of implementation hospitals have achieved and the impact on breastfeeding rates.

- The types of solid foods *first* introduced into an infant's diet during weaning.

- Awareness of Healthy Start as well as eligibility and registration. Also details of products exchanged for vouchers and awareness/usage of vitamins available under the scheme.

- Awareness of recommendations about vitamin supplementation in addition to folic acid and the uptake of specific vitamin supplements recommended by Health Departments.

- The nature and source of advice received on vitamin supplements, particularly vitamin D and any influences on choices to supplement.

- Whether folic acid supplements are taken pre- or post-conceptionally.

1 Introduction

11.   The 2005 Infant Feeding Survey was the seventh national survey of infant feeding practices to be conducted by BMRB Social Research on behalf of the four United Kingdom Health Departments. The latest survey was also the first for which a large enough sample existed to provide separate estimates for all four countries, as well as estimates for the UK as a whole.

12.   The main aim of the survey was to provide national estimates on incidence, prevalence and duration of breastfeeding as well as to provide data on the age of solid introduction and weaning practices until the age of 10 months. Areas covered by the survey included:

- influences on the choice of feeding method and on the duration of breastfeeding;

- the age of introduction of solid foods, and weaning practices at different ages and the relationship between these and regional and socio-economic factors;

- the impact of influences (i.e. peers, family, voluntary groups, professionals etc) on breastfeeding;

- smoking and drinking behaviours of mothers before, during and after pregnancy

13.   The main changes made to the 2005 questionnaire compared with previous surveys were as follows:

- changes to questions on feeding behaviour to allow measurement of exclusive breastfeeding[1] at different ages;

- a greater focus on the difference between infant formula and follow-on formula and when mothers switched from one to the other;.

- new questions on how mothers prepared and stored infant formula;

- changes to the questions on receipt of welfare tokens or vouchers to reflect replacement of the Welfare Food Scheme with Healthy Start;

- revised questions on feeding in public places, which reflected the greater interest in this topic.

[1]   Exclusive breastfeeding – an infant is exclusively breastfed if he or she receives only breastmilk, but no other liquids or solids except for medicine, vitamin or mineral supplements.

14. This paper identifies some of the challenges faced with regard to infant feeding, paying attention in particular to key areas that need to be addressed by UK government. A synthesis of the key findings of the 2005 survey can be found in Appendix 1.

2 Survey Methodology

15. Sample design and fieldwork procedures of the 2005 survey were broadly similar to those used in previous surveys. However, changes to the 2005 survey included moving away from a two-stage clustered sample design to a completely unclustered sample design in England; drawing from completely separate samples for England and Wales; and not over-sampling of mothers from lower social class groups.

16. A completely unclustered sample of 19,848 births was selected from all births registered in the period August to October 2005 in the United Kingdom. Samples were designed to be representative of all births during that period. Three stages of data collection were conducted:

   • Stage 1: infants 4-10 weeks old

   • Stage 2; infants 4-6 months old

   • Stage 3: infants 8-10 months old

17. A total 9,416 mothers completed and returned all three questionnaires. Mothers were only contacted in later Stages of the survey if they had responded to the previous one, and so the effect of non-response at each Stage was cumulative. 47% of all mothers who were initially sampled responded to all three Stages of the surveys, and this ranged from 50% in both Scotland and Northern Ireland to 46% in England. Analysis of the 2005 survey showed a consistently lower response rate in all countries among younger mothers and in areas of higher deprivation at all Stages of the survey. However, all data were weighted to correct for differential sampling and for differential response rates among different groups.

18. In addition, since previous surveys have shown the incidence of breastfeeding is strongly associated with age and educational level of the mother, incidence figures were standardised to assess the extent to which any increase in the incidence of breastfeeding in this period was attributable to demographic

changes in the sample, as opposed to a 'real' increase. Although data for incidence of breastfeeding were standardised in this way, adjustment was not made to the remaining data.

3 UK infant feeding strategy

19.   An extensive body of scientific evidence supports the consensus that *not* breastfeeding increases the risk of illness in both mothers and infants. Formula-fed babies are more likely to develop a number of conditions including gastrointestinal, respiratory and urinary tract infections (Horta et al, 2007; Ip et al, 2007). Babies who are not breastfed are also more likely to be hospitalised as the result of infection (Quigley et al, 2007). Blood pressure, total cholesterol, the prevalence of overweight/obesity and type-2 diabetes are lower among breastfed babies (Horta et al, 2007). In addition, mothers who have not breastfed are at greater risk of some cancers in later life, particularly breast cancer and ovarian cancer. They are also less likely to return to their pre-pregnancy weight (Word Cancer Research Fund, 2007).

20.   Government policy in the UK has consistently supported breastfeeding as important in the promotion of maternal and infant health. Early in 2000, the World Health Organisation (WHO) commissioned a systematic review of the published scientific literature on the optimal duration of exclusive breastfeeding (Kramer & Kakuma, 2002) and as a result, revised its guidance in 2001 to recommend exclusive breastfeeding for the first six months of an infants' life (World Health Organisation, 2001).

21.   In 2001, the UK Scientific Advisory Committee on Nutrition (SACN) considered this revised recommendation and concluded that there was sufficient evidence at the population level to advise that exclusive breastfeeding for six months is nutritionally adequate. From 2003 onwards, UK Health Departments adopted this revised guidance. The current infant feeding recommendations are as follows (Department of Health, 2003b):

   •   Breastmilk is the best form of nutrition for infants

   •   Exclusive breastfeeding for the first six months of an infant's life

   •   Six months is the recommended age for the introduction of solids for infants

   •   Breastfeeding (and/or infant formula, if used) should continue beyond the first six months, along with appropriate types and amounts of solid foods

22.   In 2003, to strengthen world attention to the impact that infant feeding practices have on the nutritional status, growth and development, health, and thus the very survival of infants and young children, the *Global Strategy for Infant and Young Child Feeding* was developed (World Health Organisation, 2003).

23.   In order to support and promote the current infant feeding recommendations, a range of measures and initiatives have been undertaken across the UK. In particular, several governmental, professional and non-governmental initiatives have been established in the UK in an effort to increase the proportion of women both initiating and maintaining breastfeeding.

24.   A Joint Breastfeeding Initiative was set up in 1988 in England and Wales, by the Department of Health, to encourage a closer working relationship between health professionals and voluntary organisations promoting breastfeeding. A similar initiative known as the Scottish Joint Breastfeeding Initiative was set up in Scotland in 1990.

25.   National Breastfeeding Awareness Week, co-ordinated in England by the Department of Heath, is a nationwide campaign that takes place each year. This annual campaign aims to raise public awareness about the benefits of breastfeeding by producing a range of engaging materials and undertaking media activity.

26.   Healthy Start, which replaced the Welfare Food Scheme (WFS) in November 2006, is a government initiative that aims to help eligible families from low-income and disadvantaged households, in England, Scotland, Wales and Northern Ireland, by giving vouchers for free milk and fresh fruit and vegetables to parents of young children and pregnant mothers. The scheme encourages earlier and closer contact with health professionals who can give advice on pregnancy, breastfeeding and healthy eating. Free vitamin supplements remain an important part of the new scheme, with new Healthy Start branded supplements made available to mothers and babies through the NHS.

27.   In 1992, the Baby Friendly Hospital Initiative, a worldwide WHO/UNICEF initiative was introduced to improve support for breastfeeding during maternity care and to encourage maternity hospitals to implement the *Ten Steps to Successful Breastfeeding* (UNICEF, 2001). The Initiative works with the health care system to ensure a high standard of evidence-based care for

pregnant women, mothers and babies. The Baby Friendly Initiative (BFI) came to the UK in 1994 and there are now 132 UK maternity hospitals with full Baby Friendly accreditation[2] or a Certificate of Commitment[3]. Of these, 51 maternity hospitals hold full accreditation. In England, only 11% of births occur in Baby Friendly hospitals, compared to 39% in Northern Ireland, 58% in Scotland and 46% in Wales (http://www.babyfriendly.org.uk).

28.   In addition to UK wide activities, each country has also developed its own specific strategy and activities for promoting breastfeeding and guidance and advice on infant feeding.

England

29.   In 1999, an Infant Feeding Initiative was launched in England to increase the incidence and duration of breastfeeding amongst those groups of the population least likely to breastfeed, as part of the government commitment to improving health inequalities. Two national infant feeding advisers were appointed to provide an infrastructure for the development and dissemination of strategies for promoting breastfeeding. Over the three-year project, money was allocated from the Public Health Development Fund to support projects that identified and developed innovative practices that aimed to increase breastfeeding initiation and duration rates; seventy-nine proposed projects were successful in obtaining funding (Department of Health, 2003a).

30.   The NHS Priorities and Planning Framework 2003-06 contains a target to deliver an increase in breastfeeding initiation rates by two percentage points per year, with particular focus on women from disadvantaged groups. This target has been included into Local Delivery Plans, to support the Public Service Agreement (PSA) target on infant mortality for the planning period to 2008. From 2005/06 to 2006/07, 39 out of 152 PCTs in England are reported to have achieved this target (Department of Health, 2007b).

31.   In England, the Department of Health also works in partnership with non-government (NGOs) and other organisations in delivering high standard services. For example, in order to encourage hospitals to implement BFI policies, the Department is working with UNICEF and has published a new leaflet *'Off to the best start'* to assist health professionals to implement best practice and to inform parents about breastfeeding. (see publication at www.dh.gov.uk).

---

[2]   Full Baby Friendly accreditation – This is awarded when all three stages of an assessment process have been successfully completed.

[3]   Certificate of Commitment – This is the first award, given when there is a breastfeeding policy, an action plan and a signed commitment from senior staff.

Wales

32.   In Wales, a strategy for promoting breastfeeding 'Investing in a Better Start: Promoting Breastfeeding in Wales', was published in 2001 to develop and support the work of a range of lead agencies and volunteers to increase the initiation and duration of breastfeeding (National Assembly for Wales, 2001). A National Breastfeeding Co-ordinator was appointed in 2003 and a Breastfeeding Strategy Implementation Group was also set up to identify and progress priority areas for implementation, and to engender best practice in the promotion, support and protection of breastfeeding. Task and Finish Groups have also been established to focus on specific areas of activity. In addition, leaflets and regular newsletters are produced for use by health professionals and parents.

Scotland

33.   In Scotland, there have been concerted efforts by a wide range of agencies and individuals to raise awareness of the importance of breastfeeding and appropriate infant feeding, and to increase successful uptake. The Scottish Breastfeeding Group (SBG) (now the Scottish Infant Feeding Advisory Network) was set up in 1995 as a multi-disciplinary group to help contribute to policy development and to act as a conduit for the dissemination of good practice and information on breastfeeding. A National Breastfeeding Adviser was in post from 1995 to 2005 and informed and influenced policy development, contributed to the development of resources, supported and monitored NHS Board activities, and encouraged best practice. Although this post has been vacant for a while, work has gone on to widen the remit and shape to fit with developing policy and the Scottish Government expect to appoint an Infant Nutrition Co-ordinator shortly (Scottish Executives, 2006).

34.   In March 2005, a new law was passed in Scotland, the Breastfeeding (Scotland) Act, which made it an offence to prevent or stop mothers from breastfeeding a child under the age of two years in any public place (www.scotland.gov.uk). In addition, a draft Infant Feeding Strategy for Scotland was consulted upon during 2006 and will form an integral part of the Scottish Government's next phase of food and health policy, placing increased focus on promoting maternal and infant nutrition (Scottish Executives, 2006).

Northern Ireland

35.   In 1999, the Department for Health and Social Services (DHSS) published a Breastfeeding Strategy for Northern Ireland (Department of Health and Social Services, 1999). A Breastfeeding Strategy Implementation Group was set up to provide ongoing support and direction for the implementation of the strategy, while a Regional Breastfeeding Co-ordinator was appointed in 2002 to help promote and implement the strategy. Much of the activity for promoting and supporting breastfeeding activity has been undertaken by the Health Promotion Agency for Northern Ireland and has included the development of resources for both parents and health professionals, including the development of a website for parents aimed at promoting breastfeeding.

4 Key findings from the survey

36.   The following section summarises some of the results from the 2005 Infant Feeding Survey, focusing on key findings with particular relevance to policy. A more detailed summary of the key findings is given in Appendix 1, and the full survey can be obtained from www.ic.nhs.uk/statistics. The relevant chapters from the full Infant Feeding Survey report are indicated in brackets throughout.

Incidence, prevalence and duration of breastfeeding (Chapter 2)

37.   The survey showed that breastfeeding initiation rates had increased in 2005 (76%) compared to 2000 (69%) across the UK. This was only partly attributable to changes in maternal age and educational attainment (see Table 1, Appendix 1). The standardised figures show the greatest increase in incidence of breastfeeding initiation between 2000 and 2005 was in England and Wales, an increase from 62% to 67% respectively (Figure 1).

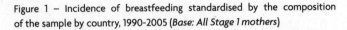

Figure 1 – Incidence of breastfeeding standardised by the composition of the sample by country, 1990-2005 (*Base: All Stage 1 mothers*)

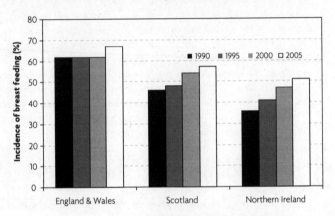

38. The prevalence and duration of breastfeeding also increased across the UK with the greatest increases seen in older mothers, mothers from higher socio-economic groups and mothers with higher educational profiles.

Figure 2 – Prevalence of breastfeeding at ages up to 9 months, United Kingdom 1990-2005 (Base: All Stage 3 mothers)

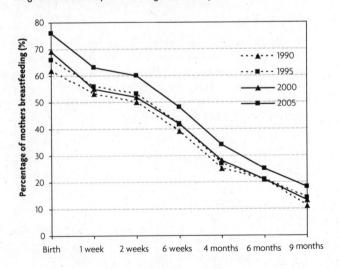

39. In addition, 45% of mothers were exclusively breastfeeding at one week, dropping to less than 1% at six months. Of mothers exclusively breastfeeding at birth, 64% lost their exclusivity[4] by giving their baby infant formula, while only 10% lost their exclusive feeding status through the introduction of solids. The latter group had fed exclusively for much longer than mothers who first introduced infant formula or other liquids.

Introduction of solids (Chapter 7)

40. The survey shows progress in delaying appropriately the introduction of solid foods. Only a very small proportion of mothers followed advice to delay introduction of solids until around six months (Figure 3).

Figure 3 – Proportion of mothers introducing solids during different age periods by survey year (1990 & 1995 Great Britain; 2000 & 2005 United Kingdom) (Base: All Stage 3 mothers 1990-2005)

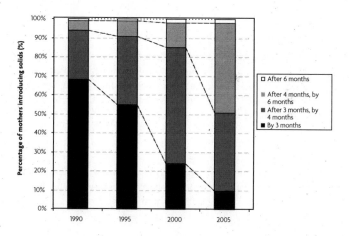

41. Inappropriately early introduction of solids was associated with receipt of advice from informal sources and tended to involve greater use of commercially-prepared foods. A higher proportion of mothers were appropriately avoiding salt, nuts, sugar, eggs and honey in their babies' diets and were more aware of food allergies compared with the 2000 survey.

---

[4] Exclusivity is considered to be lost the first time that formula or other milk, solids, or any other liquid is given to a baby.

Use of breastmilk substitutes (Chapter 5)

42. 24% of mothers in the UK did not initiate breastfeeding at birth and used infant formula as the sole source of nutrition for their baby, fewer than the 30% of mothers solely giving infant formula in 2000. By the age of six weeks, 75% of all infants were given infant formula, rising to 92% by six months.

43. At Stage 3, about half of all mothers had given their baby follow-on milk, although most mothers had followed the recommendation not to introduce follow-on milk before six months.

44. Key recommendations for preparing and storing infant formula issued by UK Health Departments and the Food Standards Agency (FSA) were commonly not adhered to. Only 13% of mothers followed all three recommendations of making one feed at a time, making feeds within 30 minutes of the water boiling, and pouring the required amount of water into the bottle before adding the powder.

Use of dietary supplements (Chapter 10)

45. 79% of mothers in the UK reported that they knew why increasing folic acid in the early stages of pregnancy was recommended and 83% all mothers reported taking some action to increase their folic acid intake. There was a clear association between mothers' awareness of the recommendation for folic acid and action taken during pregnancy.

46. Over half of all mothers took some form of vitamin or mineral supplements (apart from folic acid) during their pregnancy, with 46% taking iron as either a single supplement or in combination with vitamins. At Stage 1, 33% of all breastfeeding mothers were taking vitamin or iron supplements, falling to 28% by Stage 2 and 23% by Stage 3. The most commonly taken supplements were combined multi-vitamin and iron supplements.

47. Only 3% of babies aged four to ten weeks were being given vitamin supplements, and this increased to 7% by the age of eight to ten months. The 7% of mothers giving supplements at Stage 3 had fallen from 10% in 2000.

The following sections consider key findings from the survey and identify implications for policy and future practice. It is necessary to acknowledge the observational nature of such an analysis and not to

overlook the possibility of confounding factors which may influence comparisons, and which in most cases are not adjusted for. Again, the relevant chapters from the full Infant Feeding Survey report are indicated in brackets throughout the text.

5 Inequalities in infant feeding

48. As previously mentioned, the 2005 survey showed a consistent pattern in variation of infant feeding practices according to certain socio-demographic characteristics of the mother. Younger mothers, mothers from lower socio-economic groups and mothers with lower educational levels appeared least likely to initiate and continue breastfeeding. Mothers from these groups were also more likely to introduce solids, follow-on formula and additional drinks at an earlier age. In addition, these mothers were less likely to attend antenatal check-ups and classes, or use dietary supplements.

49. Many young mothers lack access to key sources of information and advice on infant feeding such as antenatal classes, peer support programmes, friends, family and other social support networks. Although many women have access to community midwives after discharge from hospital, young first time mothers in particular may not ask for information or advice on issues such as breastfeeding. Social policies affecting educational attainment may also be important factors in feeding practices and breastfeeding rates may be influenced by health education specifically or by more general levels of schooling among mothers.

50. Research suggests that young women from low-income areas are least likely to breastfeed for a number of reasons including embarrassment, lack of role models, fear of pain, misconceptions that their baby will not gain sufficient weight from breastfeeding alone, and exposure to a bottle feeding culture, which promotes the use of artificial milk (Shaw et al, 2003).

51. The provision of tokens for free formula-milk (under the Welfare Food Scheme (WFS) at the time of the 2005 survey) may have also been a disincentive for young and low-income mothers to breastfeed their infants. A review of the WFS concluded that the scheme in place offered no material incentive for mothers who chose to breastfeed, as the retail value of the formula allocation exceeded that of liquid milk they receive (Department of Health, 2002). In November 2006

the WFS was replaced by "Healthy Start", a scheme which offers beneficiaries opportunities to exchange vouchers for fruit and vegetables as well as milk or infant formula. This treats breastfeeding and non-breastfeeding mothers more equitably and so addresses perceived disincentives to breastfeed. The effect of this on breastfeeding rates could potentially be reflected in future surveys.

Implications for policy and practice

52. Young mothers and those from lower socio-economic groups appear least likely to adopt recommended infant feeding practices, which contributes to inequalities in health and perpetuates the deprivation cycle. Infant feeding policy, as it does already, should continue targeting these groups and the profiles of such policies should be raised.

53. There is also a need to train health professionals and peer supporters to meet the needs of young and low-income mothers, and address the misconceptions they hold about breastfeeding. Raising the profile of Healthy Start's commitment to provide nutrition education and information, requires acknowledgement of training and delivery needs, particularly among health professionals and volunteers working with these vulnerable groups.

6 Findings relevant to the promotion and support of breastfeeding

54. Breastfeeding initiation rates in the UK are among the lowest in Europe and despite an increase since 1985, there is a fall in the proportion who continue. Reasons for this are multifaceted and include the influence of society and cultural norms, the organisation of health services and the lack of preparation of health professionals and others to support breastfeeding effectively.

Awareness of the health benefits of breastfeeding and intention to breastfeed

55. Mothers who said they were aware of the health benefits were more likely to initiate breastfeeding, suggesting that awareness of the health benefits might be a motivating factor in encouraging mothers to breastfeed (Chapter 3.3).

56. The survey also showed that mothers who intended to breastfeed only, did so for longer compared to mothers who said they intended to use mixed breast

and formula feeding. Mothers who said they had not intended to breastfeed but who did so initially, breastfed for the shortest time (Chapter 3.1).

Implications for policy and practice

57.   Mothers need to make an informed decision about infant feeding. A mother's intention to breastfeed is associated with awareness of the health benefits of breastfeeding and it is important to increase awareness among all mothers.

58.   There is a need to focus on the provision of education for mothers. It should be the responsibility of all health professionals and peer supporters who come into contact with the mother, to offer routinely and proactively an appropriate mix of informal, practical breastfeeding education which spans the antenatal and postnatal periods.

Problems experienced with breastfeeding

59.   The reasons mothers gave for abandoning breastfeeding suggest that relatively few mothers truly chose not to breastfeed. Three-quarters of breastfeeding mothers who gave up during the survey period said they would have preferred to breastfeed for longer (Chapter 6.3) had they been able. These findings suggest that most women who start to breastfeed are committed to it but stop because they encounter problems and find that skilled support is not readily available.

60.   Many mothers experienced problems breastfeeding in the early weeks. Without advice and support from health professionals, these mothers were less likely to continue breastfeeding their babies. The most common reasons given by mothers for stopping in the first two weeks were the baby not sucking/ rejecting the breast, having "insufficient milk" and having painful breasts or nipples. In the second week mothers also said this was because breastfeeding took too long/was tiring (Chapter 4.3). Mothers experiencing such problems may not have access to adequate practical support and advice from health professionals. Consequently, they are obliged to provide infant formula as an alternative source of nutrition for their babies. Of those who stopped in the first two weeks, 91% said they would have preferred to breastfeed longer.

Implications for policy and practice

61.   These findings emphasise the importance of providing much more skilled support for breastfeeding mothers, particularly during the early weeks, to support their choices and ensure they can breastfeed for as long as they wish. Adequate breastfeeding-specific, practical and problem solving support must be provided, preferably proactively, soon after birth.

Antenatal care and support

62.   Attending antenatal care is also related to breastfeeding outcome in the UK. Mothers who attended antenatal check-ups were more likely to initiate breastfeeding than those who had not and nearly all mothers who had discussed feeding at antenatal check-ups had discussed feeding with a midwife. Others who had advised included health visitors and doctors, indicating that all health professionals who have contact with the mother need essential skills and training to advise mothers and support them in making informed decisions (Chapter 3.6).

63.   Attendance at antenatal classes with talks or discussions on feeding appeared to have a positive relationship with a mother's intention to breastfeed, and thus on breastfeeding initiation. Only a third of mothers had attended antenatal classes, and only a third of those who had discussed feeding intentions there. In addition, antenatal classes are not well attended by women in deprived areas; barriers for many may include cost, timing, location or unavailability of classes in their area (Chapter 3.6). This could partly explain lower breastfeeding initiation rates among these groups.

Implications for policy and practice

64.   The survey findings agree with other evidence showing that attendance at antenatal classes and discussion of feeding influences a mother's feeding choice and the likelihood of breastfeeding initiation. This emphasises the importance of antenatal support for all mothers.

65.   More extensive implementation of antenatal care is required and antenatal education should include discussions on the benefits of breastfeeding, positioning and attachment for breastfeeding, and how to fit breastfeeding into everyday life. Providing better access to antenatal support for all mothers should be encouraged in order potentially to increase breastfeeding initiation and continuation rates. Promotion of antenatal care should be directed

particularly towards those mothers who are disadvantaged and less aware of the health risks associated with not breastfeeding, and to the health professionals that come into contact with them.

Maternity experience and postnatal support

66. Skin-to-skin contact with babies within the first hour of birth was also associated with breastfeeding initiation rates, higher rates being observed among mothers who had early skin-to-skin contact. Facilitating close contact between mother and baby thus seems important for successful breastfeeding initiation (Chapter 4.1).

67. Delays in initiation of breastfeeding were linked with early cessation; mothers who initiated breastfeeding after a delay of more than twelve hours were more likely to have given up in the first two weeks than mothers who initiated breastfeeding immediately or within the first few minutes (Chapter 4.2). This suggests that encouraging mothers to breastfeed soon after birth could contribute to the proportion of mothers continuing to breastfeed for longer.

68. Co-sleeping also tended to be associated with breastfeeding. Breastfeeding mothers were more likely to allow their baby to sleep in the bed at least occasionally compared with mothers giving infant formula (Chapter 4.5). Mothers need to be encouraged to adopt safe co-sleeping practices.

Implications for policy and practice

69. Giving health professionals the right skills to support breastfeeding in hospital and at home is essential to making progress on increasing initiation rates. All health professionals who come into contact with mothers and babies should have some form of breastfeeding management training, and this should focus on training professionals to provide guidance to mothers on hospital practice, especially at birth and immediately after birth.

70. The National Institute for Health and Clinical Excellence (NICE) has published best practice guidelines on postnatal care which cover the core care that every healthy woman and healthy baby should be offered during the first six to eight weeks after the birth (National Institute for Health and Clinical Excellence, 2006). The guideline sets out evidence-based advice that healthcare professionals can give parents about a wide range of issues including breastfeeding and how to deal with common health problems. All health professionals should be made aware of these guidelines.

71.   Encouraging the adoption of new practices in more maternity units such as enabling skin-to-skin contact between mother and baby immediately after birth, ensuring unrestricted breastfeeding from birth onwards and unrestricted mother-baby contact is likely to encourage better feeding practices and have a great impact on the initiation of breastfeeding.

72.   It is essential that appropriate education and training on co-sleeping be provided to all health professionals, in order that they can provide parents with accurate information about the associated benefits and risks. This will enable mothers to make well-informed decisions and reduce the risk of inappropriate bed-sharing in hospital and at home.

73.   Health Departments should continue encouraging all health facilities to have policies and practices that protect, promote and support breastfeeding. *The Ten Steps to Successful Breastfeeding* set out by the Baby Friendly Initiative provide a robust approach for ensuring high standards in maternity units, which includes encouraging breastfeeding initiation soon after birth and also showing mothers how to breastfeed. All maternity hospitals should be encouraged to adopt Baby Friendly practices to ensure the same standard of care is available for all women and to improve breastfeeding practices and initiation rates.

Peer influences

74.   There was a correlation between feeding practices of mothers themselves and those of their friends with babies, indicating the strength of peer influences. Breastfeeding intention and actual initiation and continuation rates were higher among mothers who had been breastfed themselves as infants, and who had friends who breastfed (Chapter 4.4). Increasing opportunity for mothers to associate with other breastfeeding mothers may help bring about the required fundamental shift in cultural values that can be passed on across the community and down the generations. Presently, the culture of bottle-feeding in some communities is very strong and in these communities, mothers and grandmothers are likely either to have bottle-fed, or to have breastfed for a short time only.

75.   Fathers, grandmothers and friends may also have an important influencing role and it is crucial that they are also made aware of the risks associated with not breastfeeding (Chapter 4.4). These influential individuals may be particularly important when targeting the harder to reach mothers; younger mothers, those less well-educated, those in disadvantaged groups and other communities with the lowest rates of breastfeeding.

Implications for policy and practice

76. Peer support programmes for mothers should be more widely offered during antenatal and postnatal periods, to provide information and listening support to those who require it. It is also important to ensure mothers are aware of the range of local support that is available to them.

77. In addition, it is important to ensure that fathers, friends, families and others supporting the mother during her maternal experience are also reached with the messages about the importance of breastfeeding.

Employment practices

78. As mentioned, the duration of breastfeeding varied by when the mother returned to work. Mothers who returned to work before their baby was six months old were more likely to have discontinued at four or six months than mothers who returned when their baby was older or who were not working at all by Stage 3 of the survey (Chapter 2.4).

79. Although the largest factor behind the cessation of breastfeeding among all mothers giving up after the early weeks was "insufficient milk", returning to work began to feature from six months as a reason for stopping breastfeeding (Chapter 6.3). Mothers who choose to return to work from maternity leave may face problems in continuing to breastfeed due to a lack of flexibility and understanding from their employer.

80. Nevertheless in 2005 the proportion of mothers mentioning return to work as a factor behind giving up breastfeeding, was lower than in the 2000 survey. This is consistent with longer maternity leave entitlements in 2005 compared with 2000, and suggests some mothers have been helped to breastfeed longer.

Implications for policy and practice

81. Women may be encouraged to delay returning to work in order to continue breastfeeding. It is nevertheless important that mothers who do return to work are enabled to continue breastfeeding through provision of adequate support from employers and colleagues. Employers should be encouraged to adopt a breastfeeding and return to work policy that positively encourages women to breastfeed in the interests of promoting their own and their babies' health.

Feeding facilities outside the home

82.   A small proportion of mothers reported facilities either to breastfeed or express milk at work, particularly where they used a workplace crèche. In addition, the survey found that access to these facilities was associated with a higher than average propensity for mothers to combine work and breastfeeding at five or six months (Chapter 9.2). Mothers choosing to return to work, were therefore more likely to continue breastfeeding if facilities at work were available, than if they were not.

83.   Half of mothers who had initiated breastfeeding had breastfed in public. These mothers were asked about their preference for: a). using special facilities such as a 'mother and baby room'; b). breastfeeding where they are but finding a quiet place to sit; or c). breastfeeding where they are without going to any special place. The survey found that the large majority of mothers preferred to make some special arrangement to feed (Chapter 9.7). In addition, nearly half of mothers who had breastfed in public reported encountering problems with finding somewhere to feed. Lack of suitable places to feed was one of the main factors reported by mothers when asked what had discouraged breastfeeding in public (Chapter 9.8).

84.   When asked, almost all mothers said that shops/shopping centres should provide facilities for feeding babies. Other locations suggested included restaurants, leisure centres and public transport (Chapter 9.9).

85.   Despite a great demand among mothers for baby feeding facilities, these facilities are not being made routinely available in the work place and in public places. This may be deterring mothers from breastfeeding.

Implications for policy and practice

86.   There are many barriers to breastfeeding outside the home and these provoke anxiety amongst mothers about feeding in public. This can make life especially restrictive and uncomfortable for mothers as breastfed babies often require feeding on demand.

87.   Breastfeeding mothers face many impediments in a society that is not always supportive. There is a need to encourage more establishments to welcome breastfeeding mothers and babies, and to provide suitable facilities that enable them to breastfeed comfortably whenever and wherever they are. This may help to encourage mothers to continue breastfeeding longer.

88. Breastfeeding mothers also need to feel confident that workplaces have policies in place and a culture that supports them and their babies at work. Employers should be encouraged to provide breastfeeding facilities in the work environment where appropriate and so far as practicable. Employers with existing policies and practices in place should be encouraged to make these better known and should be aware of the Workplace Regulations and Approved Code of Practice, which require employers to provide suitable facilities for pregnant and breastfeeding mothers to rest (Health and Safety Commission, 1996). The Health and Safety Executive (HSE) also recommends that it is good practice for employers to provide a private, healthy and safe environment for breastfeeding mothers to express and store milk http://www.hse.gov.uk/mothers/).

89. Employees should also have access to information on support that is offered by their employer, to enable breastfeeding to continue after returning to work. This might include suitable, comfortable and stress-free facilities to express and store breastmilk, and more flexible arrangements in working within time at work and in overall working hours, to give mothers the opportunity to express breastmilk or to breastfeed their baby at local childcare facilities. The Department of Health issues a leaflet containing advice on continuing breastfeeding after returning to work *'Breastfeeding and work: Information for employees and employers'* (Department of Health, 2007a) and this information should be made more widely available for those who require it.

7 Factors affecting the introduction of solids

90. At the time of the 2000 survey, mothers were recommended not to introduce solids before the age of four months. By the 2005 survey, this advice had been revised to recommend introduction of solid foods at six months of age.

91. Results reflect the recommendations prevailing at the time of the different surveys, with a marked trend towards mothers introducing solids later in 2005 compared with 2000 (Chapter 7.1). Progress in delaying the introduction of solids appears therefore to have been made, reflecting effective dissemination of advice. This encouraging move forward has been achieved despite the current labelling of weaning foods as suitable for infants from four months of age.

92.   Although a significant and marked shift over time towards later introduction of solids is clear, only 2% of mothers actually delayed introduction of solids until six months. This suggests that although advice may be reaching mothers to delay introduction, other constraints may be operating. The age of introduction, for example, was related to whether and when the mothers returned to work, with those returning after at least six months, or not returning at all, introducing solids later on average than those who returned earlier. In this circumstance, it may be that mothers are aware of the advice, but that other factors influence their decision to introduce solids, such as having to return to work (Chapter 7.1).

Professional support and guidance

93.   The survey asked mothers about any influences affecting their decision to begin weaning their baby on to solids. Later introduction of solids tended to be guided by professional advice from people such as the health visitor and written information sources, while the decision for early weaning was more likely to be based on informal and subjective advice such as whether the baby was satisfied with milk feeds (Chapter 7.4). It is vital that health professionals are aware of guidance issued on weaning and deliver this advice appropriately.

94.   The age at which babies were introduced to solids was also associated with the age at which babies were given additional drinks (including drinks such as water and juice). Mothers, who gave their babies solids at an earlier age, also gave additional drinks at an earlier age (Chapter 8.2).

Types of solids given

95.   The Department of Health recommends that babies under one year should not be given salt, sugar or honey. In addition, mothers are also advised to be cautious about the use of nuts, fish or shellfish, and eggs during weaning because of possible allergic reactions (Department of Health, 1994).

96.   Compared with the 2000 survey, higher proportions of mothers appeared to be following the advice to avoid the use of salt, nuts and honey in their babies' diets. Mothers avoiding foods gave reasons for doing so and the most common reason was a concern about allergies, as well as perception that this food was not beneficial, or that it was harmful to the baby (Chapter 7.3). These concerns therefore appear to be linked with a better awareness of the health issues associated with particular foods.

97. Advice also suggests that it is important to give home-prepared foods as part of weaning, in order to introduce the infant to a greater range of culturally appropriate flavours and textures than manufactured foods can provide. Mothers giving solids when babies were four to six months were much more likely to provide commercially-prepared foods than home-prepared, but the use of home-prepared foods increased by eight to ten months (Chapter 7.2).

Implications for policy and practice

98. Although there has already been a shift in the proportion of mothers introducing solids at a later age and this is an encouraging step forward in infant feeding policy, there is still a need to increase awareness of the recommendation to delay introduction until six months. Reviewing legislation on labelling of weaning foods to reflect this advice, could further encourage a trend towards six months exclusive breastfeeding.

99. It is also necessary to identify the reasons that some mothers introduce solids early, despite their awareness of the recommendation to wait until six months, and to provide appropriate problem-solving support which helps them.

100. Health professionals should consider infants' individual developmental and nutritional needs, whether breastfed, mixed fed or given solely infant formula milk, before giving advice to introduce solid foods. Regardless of whether babies are breastfed or mixed-fed on breastmilk and infant formula, mothers should be supported to choose suitable weaning foods and diversify the baby's diet at a developmentally appropriate pace. Where mothers choose to introduce solid foods before six months, they should be encouraged to follow existing guidance on appropriate types and amounts of first foods (Department of Health, 1994).

8 Use of liquids other than breastmilk

101. UK Health Departments recommend that babies are breastfed exclusively for the first six months of life, since breastmilk provides all the nutrients a baby needs during this period. It is also recommended that mothers continue giving their babies breastmilk or infant formula until they are at least a year old. This means that there should be no need for mothers to give their babies follow-on formula or additional drinks (including drinks such as water or juice) during this period.

102.   The difference between infant formula and follow-on formula is not always well understood. At the time of the 2005 survey, an infant formula was defined as a food, which is intended for particular nutritional use by infants in good health during the first months of life, *satisfying by itself the nutritional requirements of such infants'*. Follow-on formulas are foods also intended for nutritional use by infants in good health, but for infants aged over six months and constitute the *'principal liquid element in a progressively diversified diet'* (Infant Formula and Follow-on Formula Regulations, 1995[5]).

Use of follow-on formula

103.   Follow-on formula is casein-based, takes longer to digest and is sometimes claimed to be especially suitable for hungrier babies, although there is no evidence for this. Once a baby reaches six months old, mothers can give their infants follow-on milks, but there is no nutritional justification for this change (Department of Health, 2003b). Breastmilk and/or infant formula if used, remain adequate as the liquid portion of the weaning diet throughout infancy.

104.   By eight to ten months, half of mothers had introduced follow-on formula, although the vast majority had followed the recommendation not introduce this before six months. In addition, at this stage mothers were more likely to be using follow-on formula than infant formula as their baby's main source of milk other than breastmilk, (Chapter 5.5).

105.   Mothers from lower socio-economic groups were more likely to introduce follow-on formula at an earlier age. The survey also revealed that many mothers are unclear about the distinction between the different types of formula. A separate study commissioned by the Department of Health to explore the understanding and perceptions of infant formula and follow-on formula advertising in the UK, also showed that four in ten women who were aware of both thought there was no difference between them or did not know if there was a difference (Department of Health, 2005).

106.   At the time of the 2005 survey, the Infant Formula and Follow-on Formula Regulations 1995 proscribed advertising of infant formula but permitted promotion of follow-on formula. The packaging, branding and labelling of these products often closely resembles that of infant formulas This can be confusing and may well contribute to early introduction of follow-on formula, particularly in disadvantaged groups (Chapter 5.5).

[5]   Revised UK Infant Formula and Follow-on Formula Regulations will be coming in to force in January 2008.

Reasons for giving follow-on formula

107.   Mothers cited many reasons which included: experience of using this with previous children; they thought it was better for the baby since it provided him or her with more nutrients; and they thought the baby was still hungry after being fed infant formula

108.   The reasons mothers cited for giving follow-on formula suggest that they perceive follow-on formula to be necessary despite guidance issued. This perception may be exacerbated by recommendation from health professionals (Chapter 5.5).

109.   Mothers who had ever given their baby follow-on formula had also commonly cited advice from a doctor or health visitor as a reason (Chapter 5.5). This would suggest health professionals are recommending follow-on formula to mothers despite guidance issued by Health Departments that it offers no nutritional benefit over infant formula.

Use of additional drinks

110.   A high proportion of mothers were also giving their babies drinks additional to breastmilk or infant formula by four weeks. An even higher proportion were doing this by four months which suggests that messages about the adequacy of exclusive breastfeeding are not sufficiently reaching mothers (Chapter 8.1).

111.   The age at which mothers first gave their babies additional drinks varied according to whether or not they had breastfed initially. By one week, only 7% of mothers who had initiated breastfeeding had given their babies other drinks compared with 20% of mothers who formula fed from birth. (Chapter 8.2).

Reasons for giving additional drinks

112.   The reasons given by mothers who were giving additional drinks varied by the age at which these drinks were given. The main reasons given for when the babies were four to ten weeks were health-related such as constipation and indigestion. Amongst mothers of babies being given additional drinks after four months, a perception that the baby was thirsty was the major reason (Chapter 8.3). This may suggest that some mothers are not aware that breastmilk is the only source of food and water that most infants need until the age of six months. Such guidance needs to be emphasised.

Implications for policy and practice

113.   Mothers value advice from health professionals, and it is essential that health professionals provide guidance in accordance with Health Departments, to promote best breastfeeding practice and also avoid confusion when mothers are deciding how to feed their baby. It is important to ensure that health professionals are aware of guidance on the provision of follow-on formula and additional drinks, to enable a clear and consistent message reaches mothers, particularly with regard to stressing the nutritional adequacy of exclusive breastfeeding for the first six months of an infant's life. Guidance also particularly needs to engage with those mothers who are introducing these at an inappropriately early age, and health professionals need to be made aware of the groups with whom they particularly need to work.

114.   Both the Infant Feeding Survey and the Attitudes to Feeding survey commissioned by the Department of Health (2005) suggest that follow-on formula advertising may contribute to the low prevalence of breastfeeding observed in the UK. Mothers from lower socio-economic groups particularly appear to have less understanding of the difference between infant formula and follow-on formula. Restrictions on the promotion of follow-on formula are required to ensure that parents receive information about all breastmilk substitutes from independent health professionals rather than commercial sources. This could reduce the proportion of mothers introducing follow-on formula at an early age.

Preparation of infant formula

115.   Parents need education and support in using infant formula appropriately and safely. Failure to provide mothers with adequate information regarding bottle-feeding may result in unhygienic storage and preparation of feeds with attendant risk of infection, malnutrition, hypernatraemia and obesity. The Food Standards Agency and UK Health Departments have issued guidance for health professionals about the safe preparation, storage and handling of powdered infant formula (see guidance at www.dh.gov.uk). In addition, the Department of Health has issued a *'Bottle feeding'* leaflet for mothers with guidance on the safe preparation and storage of infant formula. This topic is also covered in the *'Birth to Five'* book also issued by the Department of Health. (see publications at www.dh.gov.uk).

116. Despite this guidance, the 2005 survey showed a high proportion of mothers do not follow guidelines for preparing infant formula, highlighting a lack of practical support available for mothers on feeding practice (Chapter 5.7). Although all health professionals receive both breastfeeding and bottle-feeding leaflets and are expected to use them at their own discretion, health professionals may not be distributing these routinely and there may be little independently produced information available to mothers who choose to bottle-feed. Alternatively mothers may not read or follow the guidance issued in these leaflets.

117. In addition to guidance issued, all infant formula products should have clear instructions on their packaging from which the mother can follow and safely prepare and store the feed. Results from the survey, however, again suggest that mothers are not following these instructions when preparing feeds and do not seem to be aware of the safety issues with preparing infant formula.

Implications for policy and practice

118. While health professionals should continue to promote and support breastfeeding, they should equally be able to advise parents and practically support formula feeding. To enable mothers to feed safely, health professionals need to have skills in the safe preparation and storage of formula and knowledge of the different types of formula available. The importance of distributing advice to mothers about correct procedures needs to be emphasised to all health professionals.

9 Use of dietary supplements

119. UK Health Departments recommend a daily dose of vitamins A, C and D for breastfed infants from six months, formula-fed infants who are over six months and taking less than 500 ml infant formula per day, and children under five years of age. In addition, 10 micrograms of vitamin D each day for pregnant and breastfeeding women and 400 micrograms of folic acid for women who may become pregnant and up until the 12th week of pregancy, is recommended. Pregnant women are also specifically recommended to avoid taking supplements with high levels of vitamin A.

120. A high proportion of women appeared to be aware of the folic acid recommendation and took action to increase their folic acid intake during pregnancy, mostly by taking folic acid supplements (Chapter 10.1). This suggests advice on folic acid supplementation is reaching more mothers, although the survey did not indicate whether these were taken pre- or post-conceptionally.

121. The survey reported over half of all mothers also took vitamin or iron supplements (not folic acid) during their pregnancy (Chapter 10.1). Despite recommendations, only a third of breastfeeding mothers were taking vitamin or iron supplements at four to ten weeks (Chapter 8.7). This suggests mothers are not aware of the recommendations or their importance, and may be unaware of the health consequences of depleted vitamin status, particularly in relation to vitamin D.

122. Although specific supplements excluding vitamin A are available for pregnant women, most on general sale contain vitamin A. Some women may be unaware of the recommendation to avoid vitamin A supplements during pregnancy and may be taking regular multivitamins containing vitamin A, unaware of the consequences of excessive intakes. However, it is not clear from the survey exactly which multivitamin supplements the women were taking.

123. Only a tiny proportion of mothers were giving their babies vitamin supplements, increasing slightly by the age of eight to ten months. The proportion of babies receiving vitamins had also decreased since 2000, suggesting that mothers are not aware of the recommendations, and their importance for the health of their babies (Chapter 8.6).

Implications for policy and practice

124. There is an apparent need to raise awareness of the importance of vitamin supplements for pregnant and breastfeeding women, and for infants. This message forms a part of Healthy Start's commitment to educate mothers and highlights the importance of raising the profile of Healthy Start to not only assist in promoting breastfeeding, but also encouraging the uptake of vitamins in the population. Health care professionals should also be encouraged to discuss the importance of vitamin supplements with mothers and advise them where and how to get suitable supplements locally.

10 Recommendations

Implications for policy and practice

125. The promotion of breastfeeding needs to be tailored according to the social group. Attempts should continue to be made to increase the awareness of breastfeeding among young and low-income mothers by discussing infant feeding during pregnancy and providing support in tackling practical barriers to breastfeeding. The profile of Healthy Start should be raised and health professionals, at every opportunity, should offer practical support and advice to those eligible for the scheme.

126. Raising awareness of the health risks associated with not breastfeeding is crucial if mothers are to make informed infant feeding decisions. An emphasis on the benefits of exclusively breastfeeding for the first six months, in conjunction with advice to delay introduction of solids until around six months is required.

127. The remarkable shift in age of introduction of solid foods, increasing from a mean age of fifteen weeks in 2000 to nineteen weeks in 2005, is encouraging. However further practical support which helps mothers to wait until six months, and an appropriate change in the labelling of weaning foods would be beneficial.

128. Inequalities in access to antenatal and postnatal care are apparent. Identifying sub-groups of women who do not use maternal health services is key to improving policy adherence. There is a need to make antenatal and postnatal services more accessible for women from hard-to-reach groups and encourage them to use these services more frequently. In addition, the topic of breastfeeding should be raised whenever possible during antenatal consultations and encouragement should focus on those least likely to breastfeed.

129. Hospitals should facilitate practices conducive to breastfeeding, such as initiating breastfeeding soon after birth and encouraging close contact between mother and baby. All hospitals should have a written breastfeeding policy that is communicated and implemented.

130. All women and their families should also be given information about availability and access of postnatal care in their local community, and health professionals

working in the community need to ensure that infant feeding advice and support is widely available for mothers who require it.

131. The Baby Friendly Initiative (BFI) sets rigorous standards for health care organisations to adopt, with the aim of improving breastfeeding rates. Further encouragement should be given to all health care providers, both hospital and community, to implement a structured programme such as the BFI, which will actively encourage breastfeeding and aim to increase breastfeeding initiation and continuation rates. All health professionals should be made aware of the NICE guidance on postnatal care, which establishes clear, much needed national standards on the support women need in the weeks following birth.

132. There is a need to encourage training of health professionals in practical management of breastfeeding support and to maintain relevant skills. In addition, it is essential to ensure there are enough trained individuals easily accessible by mothers who need this support.

133. Provision of infant feeding facilities in both work and public places should be encouraged in order to welcome breastfeeding mothers and establish breastfeeding as the norm. Facilities should include suitable, comfortable and stress-free areas to express and store breastmilk.

134. Parallel to the promotion and support of breastfeeding practices, there is a need to provide clear, independent professional advice on infant formula and follow-on formula, particularly among hard-to-reach groups of mothers. Advertising of infant formula has been proscribed in the UK for some time; the Regulations must be rigorously enforced and consideration given to restricting all other forms of marketing communication.

135. It is vital that all parents and carers who choose to give their babies infant formula are offered appropriate and tailored advice on formula feeding, to ensure this is undertaken as safely as possible. It is important that all health professionals are educated about formula feeding and can offer mothers guidance on correct preparation and storage of infant formulas, as well as independent advice, which helps them to choose from the range available.

136. All health professionals working with children, pregnant women and mothers, should as part of their training, be informed of the importance of vitamin supplementation during pregnancy and breastfeeding, particularly with regard

to vitamin D and folic acid. Health professionals should particularly encourage the uptake of Healthy Start vitamins by young mothers and those from low-income groups, and should offer guidance on vitamin supplementation to all women, including advice on suitable ways of obtaining vitamin supplements. Mothers not eligible for the scheme should also be made aware that Healthy Start vitamins are available to them at a small cost.

137. The Committee endorses the forthcoming NICE guidance for primary care on Maternal and Child Nutrition in low-income families, implementation of which should help to promote improved infant feeding practices.

Suggestions for future surveys

138. The definition of *'Breastfed initially'* as *"all babies whose mothers put them to the breast, even if this was one occasion only"* should be re-examined to clarify interpretation of the term and its implications. Future surveys might include an additional question to identify any introduction of supplementary feeding within the first 24 hours.

139. Further questions about the help and advice available to mothers throughout antenatal and postnatal periods could usefully uncover what form of advice mothers find the most useful, and which strategies are most effective in delivering messages to mothers. More specifically, details of the kind of breastfeeding support received by mothers in the community could identify forms of support which are associated with increased incidence and prevalence of breastfeeding. This would be invaluable information for increasing its provision.

140. Future surveys should attempt to obtain data on the number of babies born in Baby Friendly hospitals and the impact of this on breastfeeding rates. Information as to whether the place of birth had gained full Baby Friendly accreditation[2], a "Certificate of Commitment"[3], or implemented local policy would be useful in assessing the impact of stages in BFI implementation on breastfeeding rates.

141. Information regarding the types of solid foods *first* introduced into an infant's diet during weaning would be useful in addition to general information regarding types of solids given and avoided.

142.   Following the launch of Healthy Start, future surveys should capture more information regarding awareness of the scheme, eligibility and registration. In addition, mothers should be asked for what they exchange their vouchers, and whether they are aware of and/or use the vitamins available under the scheme. Information captured should particularly enable an assessment of Healthy Start's impact on breastfeeding rates and on uptake of vitamins by mothers in the UK.

143.   Future surveys should also capture information on the use of dietary supplements for both mothers and babies. This should include:

- Awareness of the recommendations issued by Health Departments, for vitamin supplements in addition to folic acid i.e. vitamins A and D.

- Actual uptake of vitamin supplements.

- The nature and source of advice, if any, received on vitamin supplements and recommendations, and any influences on a mother's choice to use supplements or not.

- Whether mothers taking folic acid supplements use them pre- or post conceptionally.

- What vitamins the mother is taking (i.e. Healthy Start vitamins, regular multivitamins or special multivitamins for pregnant women).

References

Bolling K, Grant C, Hamlyn B, Thornton A. (2007) Infant Feeding Survey 2005. The Information Centre

Department of Health (1994) *Weaning and The Weaning Diet.* no 45. London: HMSO

Department of Health (2002) *Scientific Review of the Welfare Food Scheme.* no. 51. London: TSO

Department of Health (2003a) Infant Feeding Initiative: A Report Evaluating the Breastfeeding Practice Projects 1999-2002. http://www.dh.gov.uk/en/Publicationsandstatistics/Publications/PublicationsPolicyAndGuidance/DH_4084457

Department of Health (2003b) Infant Feeding Recommendation http://www.breastfeeding.nhs.uk/en/docs/FINAL_QA.pdf

Department of Health (2005) Attitudes to feeding: Report of survey findings. http://www.dh.gov.uk/en/Publicationsandstatistics/Publications/PublicationsPolicyAndGuidance/DH_4118853

Department of Health (2007a) Breastfeeding and work: Information for employees and employers http://www.breastfeeding.nhs.uk/en/materialforclients/downloads/leaflet_4.pdf

Department of Health (2007b) Local Delivery Plan Healthcare Commission Indicator NHS Feedback Q4 2006/07: Mothers Initiating Breastfeeding. http://www.dh.gov.uk/en/Policyandguidance/Healthandsocialcaretopics/Maternalandinfantnutrition/DH_073254

Department of Health and Social Services (1999) Northern Ireland Breastfeeding Strategy (Belfast: DHSS) http://www.dhsspsni.gov.uk/publications/archived/breastfeeding.pdf

Health and Safety Commission (1996) Workplace health, safety and welfare. Workplace (Health, Safety and Welfare) Regulations 1992 (as amended by the Quarries Miscellaneous Health and Safety Provisions Regulations 1995): Approved Code of Practice and guidance. HSE Books

Horta, B., Bahl, R., Martines, J. & Victora, C. (2007) Evidence on the Long-term Effects of Breastfeeding: Systematic Reviews and Meta-Analysis. World Health Organisation. http://www.who.int/child-adolescent-health/New_Publications/NUTRITION/ISBN_92_4_159523_0.pdf

Infant formula and follow-on formula regulations (1995) No. 77 Statutory Instruments

Ip, S., Chung, M., Raman, G., Chew, P., Magula, N., DeVine, D., Trikalinos, T. & Lau, J. (2007) Breastfeeding and Maternal and Infant Health Outcomes in Developed Countries. Evidence Report/Technology Assessment No. 153 (Prepared by Tufts-New England Medical Center Evidence-based Practice Center, under Contract No. 290-02 0022). AHRQ Publication No. 07-E007. Rockville, MD: Agency for Healthcare Research and Quality

Kramer, S. & Kakuma, R. (2002) The optimal duration of exclusive feeding: A systematic review (Cochrane Library)

National Assembly for Wales (2001) Investing in a Better Start: Promoting Breastfeeding in Wales (Cardiff: NAW) http://www.wales.nhs.uk/publications/bfeedingstrategy-e.pdf

National Institute for Health and Clinical Excellence (2006) Postnatal care: routine postnatal care of women and their babies. Clinical Guideline 37 http://www.nice.org.uk/CG037

Quigley, M.A., Kelly, Y.J. & Sacker, A. (2007) Breastfeeding and Hospitalization for Diarrhoeal and Respiratory Infection in the United Kingdom Millennium Cohort Study. *Pediatrics* 119, e837-e842

Scottish Executive (2006) Infant Feeding Strategy for Scotland: A Consultation Paper (Edinburgh: Scottish Executive) http://www.scotland.gov.uk/Publications/2006/04/03092034/0

Shaw, R., Wallace, L.M. & Bansal, M. (2003) "Is Breast Best? Perception of infant feeding". *Community Practitioner* 76(8), 299-303.

UNICEF (2001) Implementing the Baby Friendly Best Practice Standards (London: UNICEF-UK Baby Friendly Initiative) http://www.babyfriendly.org.uk/pdfs/impguide.pdf

World Cancer Research Fund / American Institute for Cancer Research (2007) Food, Nutrition, Physical Activity, and the Prevention of Cancer: a Global Perspective. Washington DC: AICR

World Health Organisation (2001) The optimal duration of exclusive breastfeeding: report on an expert consultation. Geneva: WHO

World Health Organisation (2003) Global Strategy for Infant and Young Child Feeding. Geneva: WHO

Appendix 1:

Key findings from the survey

The following information summarises the analysis of results of the 2005 Infant Feeding Survey, focusing on findings in areas with particular relevance to policy. The relevant chapters from the full Infant Feeding Survey report are indicated.

Incidence, prevalence and duration of breastfeeding (Chapter 2)

Incidence of breastfeeding

- Initial breastfeeding rates in the UK as a whole had increased in 2005 (76%) compared to 2000 (69%). However differences in age and education level of the sample may have accounted for some of the observed increase in incidence between 2000 and 2005 (Table 1 shows data by country adjusted and unadjusted for these factors).

Table 1 - Estimated incidence of breastfeeding standardised[1] by the composition of the sample by country, 1985-2005

	1985	1990	1995	2000	2005
% who breastfed initially	%	%	%	%	%
England & Wales					
Unstandardised percentage	65	64	68	71	77
Standardised percentage	65	62	62	62	67
Scotland					
Unstandardised percentage	48	50	55	63	70
Standardised percentage	48	46	48	54	57
Northern Ireland					
Unstandardised percentage	n/a	36	45	54	63
Standardised percentage	n/a	36	41	47	51
[1] Standardised for mother's age and age finished full-time education					

(taken from Infant Feeding Survey 2005: Chapter 2 Table 2.9)

- The greatest change was seen in socially disadvantaged groups although there was still a clear association between breastfeeding and socio-economic status. Mothers from managerial and professional occupations (88%), those with the highest educational profile (91%), aged 35 and over (84%) and first time mothers (79%) had the highest incidences of breastfeeding, evident in all countries.

Prevalence and duration of breastfeeding

- Prevalence of breastfeeding increased at all infant ages up to nine months in both England and Wales and Northern Ireland, and was again highest among mothers from managerial and professional occupations (65%), with the highest educational profile (39%), aged 30 or over (36%), and from ethnic minority groups.

- Just under half of all mothers in the UK were breastfeeding at six weeks (48%), with a quarter breastfeeding at six months (25%). Mothers of second or later babies breastfed for longer than first-time babies.

Exclusivity of breastfeeding

- 45% of all mothers were exclusively breastfeeding at one week and this fell to 21% feeding exclusively at six weeks. At six months, prevalence of breastfeeding in all countries was less than 1%.

- Prevalence and duration of exclusive breastfeeding were higher at all ages up to four months among mothers from managerial and professional occupations, aged 30 or over and mothers with the highest education level. At four months, 17% of mothers aged 35 or over were still exclusively breastfeeding compared with just 3% of mothers aged under 20.

- Among mothers who breastfed exclusively initially, 64% lost their exclusivity[6] by giving their baby infant formula, while 10% lost their exclusive feeding status through the introduction of solids. Mothers who first introduced solids fed exclusively for much longer than mothers who first introduced infant formula or other liquids.

Choice of feeding methods (Chapter 3)

Planned method of feeding

- 70% of mothers in the UK reported that they intended to breastfeed, with most intending to only breastfeed rather than to mix breast and formula feeding.

---

[6] Exclusivity is considered to be lost the first time that formula or other milk, solids, or any other liquid is given to a baby.

- The proportion of mothers intending to breastfeed had risen since 2000, with mothers in England (72%), first-time mothers (73%), second-time mothers who had breastfed their previous child for six weeks or more (95%), mothers who had been breastfed themselves as infants (85%), and mothers who had friends who breastfed being more likely to intend to breastfeed (90%).

- In addition, breastfeeding mothers whose friends mostly formula-fed were more likely to have given up in the first two weeks (29%) than those whose friends mostly breastfed (9%). This association continues beyond the first fortnight with 59% of mothers with friends who mainly formula fed still breastfeeding at four weeks compared with 85% of mothers whose friends mainly breastfed.

- There was a high correlation between intention to breastfeed and actual initial breastfeeding behaviour, where almost all mothers who intended to breastfeed actually did so.

Awareness of the health benefits of breastfeeding

- 84% of mothers said they were aware of the health benefits of breastfeeding, with 80% actually being able spontaneously to give one or more specific benefit. Mothers in Northern Ireland and Scotland (88% and 87% respectively), mothers from managerial and professional occupation groups (94%) and older mothers (90%) being the most likely to be aware of the health benefits.

- Mothers who said they had intended to breastfeed only were more likely to be aware of the health benefits of breastfeeding than mothers who had planned to use infant formula only (91% vs. 69% respectively), with a similar association between level of awareness of the health benefits and actual initiation.

Sources of advice about the health benefits of breastfeeding

- Approximately 80% of mothers had received some advice during their pregnancy about the health benefits of breastfeeding, mainly via midwives who were mentioned by 87% of all mothers who had received any advice.

- Mothers receiving advice were more likely to initiate breastfeeding.

Antenatal care

- Nearly all mothers said they had attended antenatal check-ups with 68% saying they had discussed feeding intentions at these check-ups.

- Only a third of mothers had attended antenatal classes with only 28% discussing feeding intentions at these classes.

- Mothers who had attended antenatal classes where feeding was discussed or where they were taught how to position the baby were more likely to intend to breastfeed (85% and 87% respectively) than mothers who did not attend these classes (63%).

- Mothers who had never worked were much less likely to have attended antenatal classes (12%) than mothers with managerial and professional occupations (50%).

Birth, postnatal care and the early weeks (Chapter 4)

Positioning the baby

- 72% of mothers had been shown how to position and attach their baby for breastfeeding in the first few days.

- The majority (85%) of mothers who had received help or advice found this most useful if the person giving advice stayed with them until the baby had started to feed.

- Only 11% said that the person giving advice stayed until the end of the feed, while 49% said they had left once the baby was feeding but came back to check on the mother.

Feeding problems

- 33% of mothers had experienced feeding problems either in hospital or in the early weeks after leaving.

- Mothers who were giving infants a combination of breastmilk and infant formula experienced the highest levels of problems (52%).

- Problems encountered mainly concerned difficulties with attachment or failure to feed, sore nipples and unsatisfied babies.

- Over eight in ten (83%) mothers who experienced problems while in hospital were offered help or advice. After leaving hospital there was a similar level of support for mothers experiencing problems (88%).

Those who did receive help for these problems were more likely to have continued breastfeeding than those who did not receive help.

Sharing the parental bed

- Approximately half of all mothers allowed their baby to sleep in the parental bed at least occasionally and this was a regular practice for 11%.

- Co-sleeping was also particularly associated with breastfeeding mothers (61%) however, 38% of mothers feeding infant formula described this practice on occasions.

Skin to skin contact

To support the initiation of breastfeeding, the UNICEF UK Baby Friendly Initiative guidelines require hospitals to encourage mothers to hold their babies in skin-to-skin contact as soon as possible after delivery in an unhurried environment regardless of intended feeding method (UNICEF, 2001). The 2005 survey showed:

- 72% of mothers reported skin-to-skin contact with babies within an hour of the birth

- Breastfeeding initiation was much higher in this group with 87% breastfeeding within this first hour compared to only 57% breastfeeding in the first hour without skin-to-skin contact.

The use of milk other than breastmilk (Chapter 5)

Use of infant formula

- 24% of mothers in the UK did not initiate breastfeeding at birth and used infant formula as the sole source of nutrition for their baby, a reduction from the 30% of mothers solely giving infant formula in 2000.

- By Stage 1, 38% of mothers who breastfed initially used infant formula as the only source of milk, rising to 58% at Stage 2 and 78% at Stage 3.

- By the age of six weeks, 75% of all infants were given infant formula, rising to 92% by six months.

Use of follow-on formula

- At Stage 3, about half of all mothers had given their baby follow-on milk, although most mothers had followed the recommendation not to introduce follow-on milk before six months.

- The most likely mothers to say they had given follow-on milk at an earlier age were mothers from routine and manual occupations (12%), mothers who had never worked (16%) and mothers with the lowest education level (12%) who had all introduced formula by four months.

- At Stage 2 of the survey, mothers who had ever given their baby follow-on formula were asked their reasons for doing so. 23% of mothers said this was because of experience of using follow-on milk with previous children and other common reasons given were because they had been advised to by a doctor or health visitor (22%), because they thought it was better for the baby (20%) and because the baby was still hungry after being fed infant formula (18%).

- 25% of first time mothers said they had been advised by a health professional to use follow-on milk, while 24% said they thought it was better for the baby.

Preparation of infant formula

- Of artificially feeding mothers, 69% prepared several feeds at a time and stored them.

- Just under half of all mothers who had prepared powdered infant formula in the last seven days, had not followed key recommendations for preparing formula; either by not always using boiled water that had been cooled for less than 30 minutes, or not always using water to the bottle before the powder.

- Approximately one third did not follow infant formula preparation recommendations when away from home (i.e. they did not keep pre-prepared formula chilled or used cold or cooled water when preparing the feed).

- Only 13% of all mothers followed all three recommendations of only making one feed at a time, making feeds within 30 minutes of the water boiling, and adding the water to the bottle before the powder.

Feeding and health after the early weeks (Chapter 6)

Problems with feeding

- Beyond the early weeks, approximately one in eight mothers had experienced breastfeeding problems between Stages 1 and 2; and one in ten between Stages 2 and 3.

- Mothers who breastfed between Stages 1 and 2 experienced more feeding problems compared with mothers who formula fed throughout (12 - 22% vs. 7% respectively).

- The greatest incidence of problems was found amongst mothers who continued to breastfeed with introduction of supplementary formula (22%), with most common problems cited being: inability to satisfy the baby (25%), a need to top up with formula (27%) and blocked milk ducts (24%).

- Overall, the single largest factor behind breastfeeding cessation between one week and four months, was "insufficient milk", while giving up in the early weeks (weeks one and two) was more associated with rejection of the breast, and painful breasts or nipples.

Mothers' choice and breastfeeding intentions

- Nine in ten mothers who stopped breastfeeding during the first six months said they would like to have carried on longer. Although the proportion was highest in the early weeks it was still high (40%) amongst mothers who fed for at least six-months.

Support during breastfeeding

- Mothers who received help were more likely to continue breastfeeding than those who did not receive help.

Health problems with the baby

- Babies who were breastfed for at least six months were significantly less likely to suffer from colic, constipation, sickness/vomiting, diarrhoea, chest infections and thrush; and the likeliness of developing symptoms for these conditions decreased with breastfeeding duration.

Introduction of solid foods (Chapter 7)

Age of introduction of solids

- Solid food introduction was later than reported in earlier surveys, with only 51% of mothers introducing solids by four months compared to 85% in 2000, although only 2% had delayed the introduction of solids until six months.

- Solids food tended to be introduced at a younger age among mothers from Wales and Scotland (65% and 60% respectively), mothers from routine and manual occupation groups (61%) and mothers with lower educational levels (63%), who had all introduced solids by four months.

- Mothers from ethnic minority groups were more likely to introduce solids later than white mothers where 93 – 97% of mothers from ethnic minority groups had introduced solids by six months compared with 98% white mothers. Mothers who returned to work before six months were more likely to have introduced solid foods than those who had delayed their return until at least six months (56 – 59% vs. 49% respectively).

Advice on introduction of solids

- Later introduction of solids was associated with receiving advice from health professionals whereas earlier introduction of solid foods was more likely to be based on informal advice sources and subjective criteria such as whether the baby was considered to be sufficiently satisfied with milk feeds and previous experience.

Solid foods given and avoided

- Mothers giving solids when babies were four to six months old were more likely to provide commercially prepared foods than home prepared.

- A large majority of mothers (92%) avoided the use of salt in the diets of eight to ten month old babies, although mothers of the lowest occupation group (25%) and of ethnic minority backgrounds (32% Asian mothers; 26% Chinese or other; and 23% Black mothers) were more likely to "sometimes" use salt.

- A high proportion of mothers said they avoided the use of nuts, sugar, eggs and honey in their babies' diets and there was generally a greater awareness of food allergies in the 2005 survey compared with 2000.

- The principal source of advice relating to introduction of solid foods and what type of foods to give was the health visitor (87%).

Additional drinks (Chapter 8)

The introduction of additional drinks

- By four weeks, 32% of mothers in the UK had given their babies additional drinks[7] to breastmilk or infant formula, and this rose to 64% by four months and 84% by six months.

- Breastfed infants were less likely than formula fed infants to be given additional drinks.

Reasons for giving additional drinks

- At Stages 1 and 2 of the survey, common reasons given by mothers for giving additional drinks were because the baby was thirsty, to help constipation, to help colic/wind/indigestion, or to help settle their baby.

- By Stage 3, the main reason for giving additional drinks was because the baby was thirsty.

Vitamin and mineral supplements for mothers and babies (Chapter 8)

Supplementary vitamins for the baby

- Only 3% of babies aged four to ten weeks were being given vitamin supplements, and this increased to 7% by the age of eight to ten months. The 7% of mothers giving supplements at Stage 3 had fallen from 10% in 2000.

- Babies who had been in special care after birth or who were significantly underweight at birth (under 2.5kg) were more likely to be receiving vitamin supplements at all three stages.

- Asian and Black mothers (25% and 23% respectively) were more likely than white mothers to give their babies supplementary vitamins.

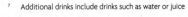

7   Additional drinks include drinks such as water or juice

Supplementary vitamins for the mother

- At Stage 1, 33% of all breastfeeding mothers were taking vitamin or iron supplements, falling to 28% by Stage 2 and 23% by Stage 3. The most commonly taken supplements were combined multi-vitamin and iron supplements.

Feeding outside the home (Chapter 9)

Feeding the baby after return to work

- By Stage 3, 45% of all mothers had returned to work, with 57% returning to work after the baby was six months old.

- Of those mothers working, 14% were working less than 15 hours per week and a further 56% working between 15 and 30 hours.

- 15% said they had facilities to either breastfeed or express milk at work, and these facilities were particularly associated with mothers using a workplace creche.

Feeding in public places

- The large majority of mothers had fed in public by Stage 2 and Stage 3, with 39% having breastfed and 67% having bottle-fed.

- By country, the prevalence of feeding in public reflected the differential breastfeeding rates by country, thus the rate of breastfeeding in public was highest in England.

- Breastfeeding in public was associated with older mothers (60%), more educated mothers (61%), and mothers with managerial and professional occupations (63%). Black mothers were also more likely to breastfeed in public (62%) than breastfeeding mothers from other ethnic backgrounds.

- 46% of all mothers breastfeeding initially said they had encountered problems finding somewhere to feed. Only 3% said they had been stopped or asked not to breastfeed in public, although 13% said they had been made to feel uncomfortable.

A new law passed in Scotland in March 2005, gave mothers the right to feed in public. Encouragingly the survey found that:

- 55% of breastfeeding mothers in Scotland said they had breastfed in public compared to other countries (40% in Northern Ireland; 44% in Wales; 52% in England).

- Breastfeeding mothers in Scotland were less likely to experience problems finding somewhere suitable to breastfeed (33%) or be stopped or made to feel uncomfortable (8%).

Dietary supplements, smoking and drinking during pregnancy (Chapter 10)

Use of folic acid supplements

- Across the UK, 79% of mothers reported that they knew why increasing folic acid in the early stages of pregnancy was recommended.

- Mothers in Northern Ireland, mothers from managerial and professional occupation groups, older mothers and mothers with the highest education level were most likely to be aware of this recommendation.

- 83% of all mothers in the UK reported taking some action to increase their folic acid intake: 75% said they had taken supplements, while 28% said they had changed their diet to eat more foods rich in folic acid.

- Mothers in Scotland and Northern Ireland (85% and 88% respectively), mothers from managerial and professional occupations (93%), and white mothers (85%) were all more likely to take action to increase folic acid intake. There was a clear association between mothers' awareness of the recommendation for folic acid and action taken during pregnancy.

Use of other vitamins and minerals

- Over half (54%) of all mothers took some form of vitamin or mineral supplements (apart from folic acid) during their pregnancy, with 46% taking iron as either a single supplement or in combination with vitamins.

Smoking during pregnancy

- 33% of mothers in the UK smoked in the twelve months before or during their pregnancy, with 48% of these mothers giving up at some point before birth. 17% of all mothers continued to smoke throughout pregnancy.

- Mothers in routine and manual occupations and those aged 20 or under were more likely to smoke before or during pregnancy and these groups were also least likely to have given up smoking at some point before or during pregnancy.

- 87% of mothers who were smoking before pregnancy received some advice or information on smoking, with midwives, books, leaflets and magazines and doctors being reported as the most common sources of information.

Alcohol consumption during pregnancy

- 54% of mothers drank alcohol during pregnancy and this was more likely among mothers from managerial and professional occupation groups and older mothers.

- The proportion of mothers drinking alcohol during pregnancy had fallen since 2000 and consumption levels were low.

49